SirtFood Manual

A quick start Guide to cooking on the SirtFood diet!
Easy and tasty recipes to burn fat and stay fit

Lisa T. Oliver

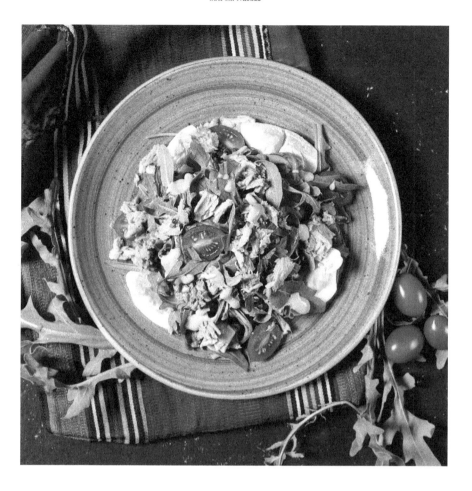

© Copyright 2021 All rights reserved.

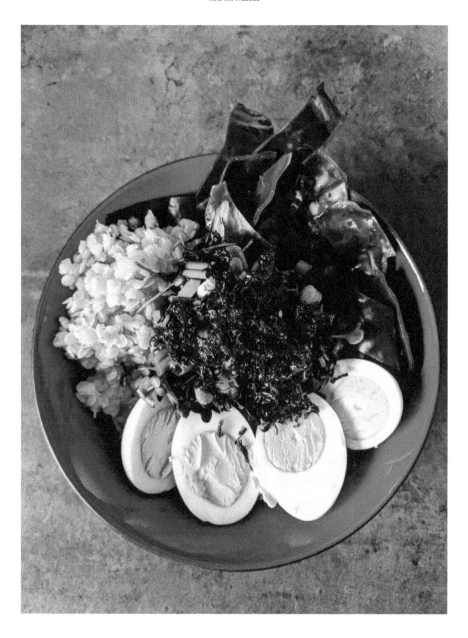

Table of Contents

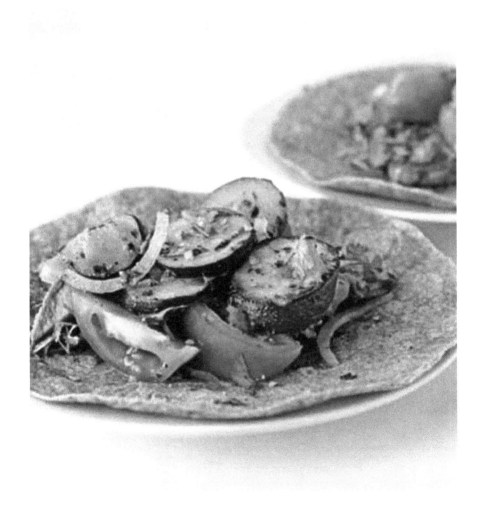

Introduction

What Are Sirtfoods?

Sirtuins refer to a protein class that has been proven to regulate the metabolism of fat and glucose. According to research, sirtuins also have a significant impact on aging, inflammation, and cell death.

By consuming foods rich in sirtuins like cocoa, kale, and parsley, you stimulate your skinny gene pathway and lose fat faster.

About the Sirtfood Diet

The Sirtfood Diet plan considers that some foods activate your "skinny gene" and can make you lose about seven pounds in about a week.Certain foods, such as dark chocolate, kale, and wine, contain polyphenols, a natural chemical that imitates exercise and fasting and affects the body. Other sirtfoods include cinnamon, red onions, and turmeric. These trigger the sirtuins' pathway and start weight loss. There is scientific evidence to support this too. The impact of weight loss is higher in the first week. The Sirtfood Diet mainly consists of plant-based foods that are rich in sirtuins to trigger fat loss. The diet is divided into two phases, which can be repeated continuously.The first phase is three days of living on 1000 calories and four days of 1500 calories with lots of green juices.

CHAPTER 1: The Premise of the Sirtfood Diet The premise of the Sirtfood Diet states that certain foods can mimic the benefits of fasting and caloric restrictions by activating sirtuins, which are proteins in the body. They range from SIRT1 to SIRT7, switch genes on and off, maintain biological pathways, and protect cells from age-related decline. Although intense calorie restriction and fasting are severe, the Sirtfood Diet inventors developed a plan with a focus on eating plenty of sirtfoods. It's a more natural way to stimulate sirtuin genes in the body, also known as skinny genes. In the process, it improves health and boosts weight loss. If you want to start the Sirtfood Diet, planning is required, and access to the ingredients needed to follow the diet correctly. There are many exciting recipes for the diet, with a variety of ingredients. However, it may often be challenging to get certain ingredients during specific seasons and times of the year. Some of these ingredients include kale and strawberries, for example. It may also be stressful to follow social events when traveling or to care for a young child. The Sirtfood Diet covers various food groups; however, dairy foods aren't included in the plan. Sirtfoods are a new diet discovery. They are rich in nutrients and capable of activating skinny genes in the body, with benefits and downsides alike. **THE SCIENCE OF SIRTUINS**

The Sirtfood diet is very famous due to its scientific benefits and amazing transformations within the body's metabolic capacities. Thousands of people have unlocked incredible and aesthetic physiques by following the Sirtfood diet. These results are not coming from word of mouth or myths attached to basic philosophies of dieting; in fact, the Sirtfood diet has a robust yet growing scientific background. The discovery of the Sirtfood diet was not an accident, but researchers found the necessary components, the polyphenols, in labs and conducted many types of research to conform to the scientific benefits of the Sirtfood diet. The primary lean gene, also known as a sirtuin, on which this dieting style got its name was first found in 1984 and not in humans but in yeasts. Polyphenol is a well-known chemical compound present in the body and acts on an essential lean gene to activate and perform fat-burning blitz inside the human body. To be very specific, Sirtfoods are those which contain high levels of a chemical compound called polyphenol. This compound is not uniformly distributed in Sirtfoods, but every Sirtfood contains specific amounts of polyphenols. The answer is straightforward yet very informative. Polyphenols are the compounds that are present naturally in Sirtfood, and many types of research conducted have confirmed that these foods have the highest impacts when losing extra pounds of fats from the body.

Polyphenols are essential precursors in the fat burning cycle of the body called lipolysis. Free fatty acids in our blood are subjected to digestion and then excretion from the body through an enzyme called lipase. Foods rich in Polyphenols cause much increase in levels of lipase enzyme and thus more fat burning blitz in the body. Polyphenols act on lipase and other fat-burning mediators by activating a particular type of gene in the body called sirtuin. This gene is the most crucial part of the Sirtfood diet because, through this gene activation, polyphenol-rich foods called the Sirtfoods act on extra stored fat in our body and engine a fat-burning cycle in our body to get rid of it. Sirtuin gene is a human gene and present in every human. It is also present in some other animals as well but in modified forms. Interestingly, the very first encounter with the sirtuin gene was in 2002 when a group of researchers found its over-activation associated with particular types of foods given to some animals. Then many studies were conducted on mice to check the efficacy of these foods and the activation of the sirtuin gene in the human body. These trials confirmed that the sirtuin gene is associated with fat loss, and Sirtfoods, which contain the maximum amount of polyphenol, are very important when undergoing a fat loss diet.

It is also fascinating to know that Sirtfoods are not very rare types of food. These foods contain a significant portion of both eastern and western diets as well as in Mediterranean diets. The Sirtfood diet consists of the top twenty foods in the world, which are considered as the basic Sirtfoods. These twenty foods contain the highest amounts of sirtuin-activating polyphenols. The levels of polyphenol are not uniformly distributed in all these foods, and some of them contain higher amounts. Moreover, different types of polyphenols are present in these Sirtfoods, which are associated with special effects on the sirtuin gene. The most important aspect of the Sirtfood diet is that it uses a variety of foods. These twenty Sirtfoods make an essential part of the Sirtfood diet so that the maximum amount of all types of polyphenols is consumed to maximize the fat burning in our body.

CHAPTER 2: **The Science Behind the Fat-Burning Benefits of the Sirtfood Diet**

The most significant benefit of the Sirtfood diet is its incredible impact on losing fats from the body. Fats are made up of fatty acids that combine to make adipocytes. These adipocytes are clusters of fatty acids, and unlike free fatty acids, adipocytes are not mostly present in the blood. They get accumulated under the skin, in muscles, and on different organs. These adipocytes combine to make adipose tissues, which are full fledge foam-shaped cluster of visible yellowish white-color fat in our body. Adipocytes are the healthiest fat cells to burn, and they must have been broken down into adipocytes and finally in free fatty acids (in reverse order of formation) to get burned from the fat-burning enzymes called the lipase enzyme. These steps are not easy as they seem, and burning extra pounds of fats can be a hard nut to crack. The most challenging step in this cycle is to break adipose tissues in adipocytes. The Sirtfoods contain high levels of polyphenols.

CHAPTER 3: **The Sirtfood Diet and Energy Cycle of the Body**

The fuel of the body is glucose, which is the most readily available nutrient in the body for energy. The glucose is broken down into energy packets called ATPs, which are produced from the power of cells called mitochondria. These energy packets are utilized to fuel the body while performing actions. High-intensity work such as exercise requires a much more significant amount of energy as compared to typing on a keyboard. The higher the intensity of work, the larger will be the needed number of ATPs. The most significant source of glucose in the body is carbohydrates, which are sugars in simpler forms. A diet rich in low glycemic carbohydrates is essential while performing high-intensity tasks. These carbohydrates are broken down into the purest form of sugar called glucose. This glucose undergoes a series of reactions called glycolysis. In this cycle, the end product is the ATPs that are stored or utilized in response to stress produced in the body. These ATPs are also crucial for fighting against the infections because the higher the level of energy in the body, the greater will be the immune response of the body. All the processes are directly proportional.

The Sirtfood diet is affluent in proteins, good fats, and low glycemic carbohydrates. All these macronutrients are essential for fulfilling the body's essential needs of energy and refueling.

CHAPTER 4: The Sirtfood Diet and Poke Hole Theory

This is by far the most valuable information about the Sirtfood diet. Very brief literature is available about the poke hole theory and its relationship with the Sirtfood diet. When a person undergoes a diet, which comprises of a calorie deficit scenario, our body takes it as a challenge and signals our mitochondria—the powerhouse of the cell to produce ATP, which are the energy packets to supply the body with instant energy. This calorie deficit scenario pokes holes in mitochondria, and thus, specific genes are activated in a cyclic manner to produce a considerable amount of energy in response to these holes in mitochondria. You can say that mitochondria get excited in response to these poked holes. A significant benefit of this cycling production of energy is the utilization of stored fats as a source of energy. When the body is not getting enough from outside sources, it becomes evident that the body must utilize its energy stores either from fat, muscles, or available glucose.

As the energy consumption is higher and calorie intake is higher when someone starts a calorie deficit diet such as the Sirtfood diet, the body acts on cyclic use of its stored fat to mobilize it in blood, and high metabolic rates due to exercise cause consumption and immediate burning of these free fatty acids in the blood. If someone consumes fat mobilizing precursors from the diet, this fat-burning mechanism can speed up too many folds.

CHAPTER 5:

Breakfast

1. Blueberry-Buckwheat Porridge

Preparation Time: 20minutes

Cooking Time: 0 minutes

Servings: 2

Ingredients

- 2/3 cup buckwheat

- 1/2 cup blueberries

- 1 ripe banana

- 1 tbsp. chia seeds

- 1 tbsp. almond butter

- 1/4 cup almond milk

- 1 tbsp. raw honey

- 1 cup of water

Directions

Soak the buckwheat in a bowl of water overnight.

When ready, drain the buckwheat and rinse well; transfer two-thirds of the buckwheat to a blender and add blueberries, banana, chia seeds, almond milk, and honey almond butter; blend until smooth and creamy. Transfer to a serving bowl and stir in the remaining buckwheat. Enjoy!

2. Cocoa Coconut Raspberry Yogurt

Preparation Time: 10minutes

Cooking Time: 10 minutes

Servings: 2

Ingredients

1 cup plain coconut yogurt

1/4 cup chopped toasted almonds

1 pint fresh raspberries

1 cup blueberries

1/4 cup cocoa powder

Directions

Divide coconut yogurt between two serving bowls and top each with toasted almonds, berries, and cocoa powder. Enjoy!

3.   Mango, Almond & Chia Seed Breakfast Bowl

Preparation Time: 10 minutes

Cooking Time: 0 minutes

Servings: 2

Ingredients

2 tablespoons chia seeds

1/4 cup rolled oats

1 cup of soy milk

1/2 teaspoon cinnamon

2 tablespoons toasted almonds

1 mango, diced

1/3 cup natural soy yogurt

1 teaspoon cinnamon

Directions

In a bowl, mix chia seeds and oats; stir in soy milk and cinnamon until well, and refrigerate, cover, and overnight. When ready to serve, divide the oat mixture between two bowls and top each with toasted almonds, mango, and yogurt; sprinkle with cinnamon, and enjoy!

Nutrition: Energy (calories): 242 kcal Protein: 16.25 g Fat: 8.03 g Carbohydrates: 36.86 g

4. Healthy Muesli With Caramelized Apple

Preparation Time: 10 minutes

Cooking Time: 5 minutes

Servings: 6

Ingredients

- 1 1/2 cups apple juice

- 2 cups rolled oats

- 1 tablespoon raw honey

- 1/2 cup nonfat Greek yogurt

- 1/4 cup chopped toasted almonds

- 125g blueberries, chopped

- 1 apple, grated

- 1 cup Greek yogurt

- Handful of strawberries

Caramelized apple

- 1 tablespoon butter

- 1 tablespoon raw honey

- 1 apple, peeled, sliced

Directions

Stir together apple juice and oats in a bowl; chill, covered, overnight.

Melt butter in a pan and stir in raw honey and apple; cook, stirring, for about 5 minutes or until apple is caramelized.

Remove oat mixture from the fridge and stir in raw honey, yogurt, almonds, blueberries, and apple. Serve in a bowl topped with yogurt, more strawberries, and caramelized apple. Enjoy!

5.   Matcha Granola With Blueberries

Preparation Time: 15 minutes

Cooking Time: 1 hour and 15 minutes

Servings: 8

Ingredients

3 cups rolled oats

2 tbsp. extra virgin olive oil

2½ tsp. matcha powder

1 cup dried blueberries

2 cups nuts

2 tsp. vanilla extract

2 tbsp. + 1 tbsp. raw honey

¼ cup brown sugar

Big pinch of salt

Directions

Preheat your oven to 250° F.

Combine oats, sugar, and nuts in a large bowl.

In a separate bowl, combine honey, oil, vanilla, and salt; pour over the oats mixture and toss until well coated. Spread the granola mixture onto a large baking sheet and bake in the preheated oven for about 75 minutes, stirring every 15 minutes.

Put it out from the oven and scrape the mixture into the large bowl. Let it cool for a few minutes, then sprinkle matcha over and toss it. Add in dried blueberries and toss to combine.

Keep in an airtight container for a few weeks.

Nutrition:

Energy (calories): 3313 kcal

Protein: 71.96 g

Fat: 235.74 g

Carbohydrates: 369.89 g

6.   Overnight Pumpkin Oats

Preparation Time: 5 minutes

Cooking Time: 0 minutes

Servings: 4

Ingredients

1 cup rolled oats

1 ½ cups of almond milk

1/3 cup pumpkin puree

3 dates, chopped

3 tablespoons chia seeds

1 teaspoon vanilla

2 teaspoons cinnamon

1/4 cup chopped walnuts

Directions

Mix all ingredients in a mason jar; let sit overnight, stirring severally.

Serve in the morning topped with toasted walnuts.

Nutrition:

Energy (calories): 850 kca Protein: 33.92 g Fat: 43.38 g

Carbohydrates: 125.18 g

7.   Healthy Cacao Fruit Smoothie

Preparation Time: 5 minutes

Cooking Time: 0 minutes

Servings: 1

Ingredients

- 1 tablespoon peanut butter

- 1 cup coconut yogurt

- 1/4 cup blueberries

- 1 banana

- 1 tablespoon cacao powder

- 1 tablespoon chia seeds

Directions

Blend all ingredients in a blender until very smooth. Enjoy!

Nutrition:

Energy (calories): 148 kcal

Protein: 3.29 g

Fat: 3.57 g

Carbohydrates: 27.01 g

8.   Chia Seed Lime Mango Pudding

Preparation Time: 15 minutes

Cooking Time: 0 minutes

Servings: 8

Ingredients

- 3 cups fresh mango chunks

- 2 cups soy milk

- ¼ cup freshly squeezed lime juice

- 1 tablespoon lime zest

- ¼ cup raw honey

- ¼ cup hemp seeds

- ⅓ cup chia seeds

- Toasted chopped walnuts for topping

- Mango, diced, for topping

Directions

Blend mango chunks, soy milk, lime juice, lime zest, and raw honey until very smooth; add hemp and chia seeds and pulse to combine well.Refrigerate for at least 4 hours before serving.

Nutrition:Energy (calories): 1768 kcal Protein: 37.53 g Fat: 106 g Carbohydrates: 199.3 g

9.   Healthy Green Chia Pudding

Preparation Time: 90 minutes

Cooking Time: 0 minutes

Servings: 1

Ingredients

- 1 cup fresh kale

- 1 cup of soy milk

- 1 date

- 3 tablespoon chia seeds

- 1 kiwi and handful blueberries, for topping

Directions

Blend kale, soy milk, and date until smooth; transfer to a bowl and stir in chia seeds. Chill for at least 1 hour.

To serve, stir in the top with kiwi and berries.

10.   Healthy Coconut & Carrot Breakfast Bowl

Preparation Time: 5 minutes

Cooking Time: 0 minutes Servings: 2

Ingredients

- ½ cup carrot juice

- 1 cup of soy milk

- 4 tablespoons oats

- 3 tablespoons chia seeds

- 1 teaspoon cinnamon

- 1 teaspoon turmeric

- 1 teaspoon raw honey

- 1 tablespoon walnut butter

- 1 apple, sliced

Directions

In a large bowl, stir together carrot juice, soy milk, oats, chia seeds, turmeric, and cinnamon until well combined; refrigerate for at least 8 hours.To serve, stir in raw honey, walnut butter, and apple slices until well combined. Enjoy!

Nutrition:Energy (calories): 451 kcal Protein: 10.1 g Fat: 18.67 gCarbohydrates: 74.55 g

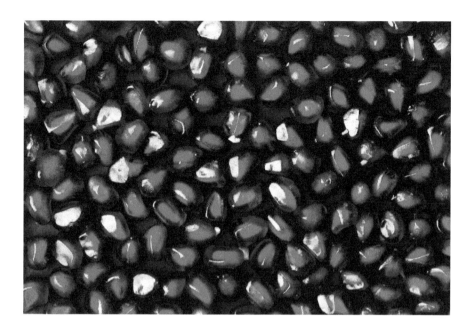

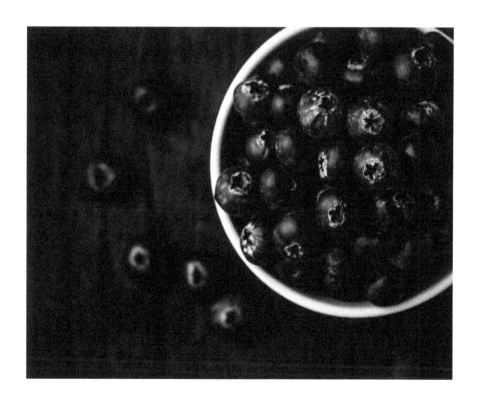

CHAPTER 6:

Lunch

11.   Stall With Pimento Cheese And Zucchini

Preparation Time: 10 minutes

Cooking Time: 15 minutes

Servings: 4

 Ingredients

2nd Tsp. olive oil

2nd Knife sp. cumin

120 Grams of zucchini (sliced lengthways)

1Slice of bread (BRIGITTE balance bread, 60 g)

40 Grams of sour milk cheese (e.g., Harzer, Mainzer)

2nd Spring onions (in rings)

Paprika powder (spicy)

40 Grams of low-fat curd

Teaspoons of orange juice

0.25 Tsp. black pepper

0.5 Handful of lettuce (e.g., lettuce)

30th Grams of tomato (pickled, semi-dried, from a glass, in strips)

Directions:

Heat a pan. Add olive oil and cumin. Add zucchini and fry briefly on both sides. Take out and let cool—toasting bread.

Dice the cheese and mix with spring onions, paprika powder, curd cheese, orange juice, and pepper.

Top the bread slice with the salad and pimento cheese and serve with zucchini and tomatoes.

Nutrition:

435 kcal,

14g fat,

43g carbohydrates,

29g protein

12.   Fish Balls, Pak Choi, And Lemon Kefir

Preparation Time: 10 minutes

Cooking Time: 40 minutes

Servings: 4

Ingredients:

250 Grams of the cod fillet (skinless)

2nd Tbsp. hemp seeds (peeled)

0.5 Tsp. fish spice (e.g. . .” Ahoi" from Herbaria)

3rd Tablespoons corn (canned corn kernels)

2nd Spring onions (finely chopped)

1 Organic lemon

4th tsp. rapeseed oil

200 Grams of pak choi (halved lengthways)

150 Milliliters of vegetable broth

75 Grams of beetroot (pre-cooked, vacuum-packed, or glass, in pieces)

80 Grams of kefir (or plain yogurt)Tbsp. mustard (sweet)salt

Directions:

Pat well-chilled fish fillet dry and dice. Puree the fish, hemp, and spice mixture. Stir in the corn kernels, spring onions, and 1–2 teaspoons of grated lemon zest. Then shape six bulbs with wet hands and chill for 10 minutes.

Spread the bottom of a hot, coated pan with two teaspoons of rapeseed oil. Briefly fry the pak choi with the cut side down, turn and add 4–6 tablespoons of vegetable stock. Cover and cook Pak Choi covered for 4–5 minutes. Add the beetroot and heat briefly.

Fry the cutlets in another pan in 2 teaspoons of hot rapeseed oil for 3 minutes over medium heat.

Mix the kefir, mustard, one pinch of salt, four tablespoons of vegetable broth, two teaspoons of grated lemon peel, and 1–2 tablespoons of lemon juice.

Arrange three fish buns with pak choi, lemon kefir, and lemon slices. Eat or freeze the remaining cutlets the next day.

Nutrition:

475 kcal,

25g fat,

25g carbohydrates,

35g protein

13.　Artichoke Salad With Caper And Egg Sauce

Preparation Time: 10 minutes

Cooking Time: 30 minutes

Servings: 2

Ingredients

A Glass of artichokes

4th Handful of leaf lettuce (seasonal leaf lettuce, e.g., lettuce and endive salad)

2nd Peppers (grilled peppers, glass, 100 g)

2nd Tablespoons chives (rolls)

60 Grams (whole grain chips)

CAPER EGG SAUCE

3rd Organic eggs

2nd Tablespoons capers (fine, glass)

2nd Tarragon mustard

2nd Tablespoons salad cream (organic)

Tablespoons apple cider vinegar (mild)

Cayenne pepper

Lemon juice

salt

Directions:

Drain the artichokes and collect the oil. Clean salad, rinse, dry, pluck into pieces. Dry and dice the grilled peppers.

FOR THE SAUCE

Boil the eggs for 7–9 minutes. Drain the capers.

Rinse eggs cold, peel, halve, and different protein and yellow. Dice the egg whites, mash the egg yolks with a fork, and mix with the mustard, lettuce cream, two tablespoons artichoke oil, and vinegar. Add 2-3 tablespoons of water after consistency. Stir in the capers, season with cayenne, possibly lemon juice, and salt.

Arrange the leaf lettuce, artichokes, peppers, and egg whites, and then pass in chips.

Nutrition:

350 kcal,

17g fat,

25g carbohydrates,

21g protein

14.   Sirt Food Smoothie After Goggins And Mats

Preparation Time: 10 minutes

Cooking Time: 30 minutes

Servings: 1

Ingredients:

100g unsweetened Greek yogurt

Six walnut halves

8-10 medium-sized strawberries

a handful of kale leaves without woody parts

20g dark chocolate (at least 85% cocoa)

1date

1/2 teaspoon of turmeric

1to 2 mm from a Thai chili, finely chopped

200ml unsweetened almond milk

Directions:

If you want it vegan, use soy yogurt instead of Greek yogurt.

Put everything in a blender or blender and mix until a smoother smoothie is made.

Tip: if I have parsley stalks left over, I still add them, chop them roughly beforehand.

More smoothies that go well with the sirt food diet or that you can drink.

Nutrition:

380 kcal

41 g protein

17 g fat

12 g carbohydrates

15.   Sirt Food Green Juice

Preparation Time: 10 minutes

Cooking Time: 15 minutes

Servings: 2

Ingredients:

Two big hands of kale

A large handful of arugula

A tiny hand of flat-leaf parsley

a small hand lovage leaves

2-3 stalks of celery, including the leaves

1/2 small green apple - e.g., Granny Smith

Lemon Juice from Half of a lemon

Half of the teaspoon of matcha powder

Directions:

First, mix the kale, rocket, parsley, and lovage and add to the juicer. About 50ml should come out. Then we recommend juicing the apple and celery stalks and squeezing half the lemon by hand. Then you should have about 250ml of liquid.

Add a small amount of this to the glass from which you will later drink and dissolve the matcha powder in it. Once it has dissolved, add the rest of the liquid.

Nutrition:

270 kcal

9 g protein

18 g fat

12 g carbohydrates

16.   Spinach Flan With Tomato Ragout

Preparation Time: 10 minutes

Cooking Time: 60 minutes

Servings: 4

Ingredients:

FLAN

250 Grams of frozen leaf spinach (thawed)

1Clove of garlic (crushed)

1 Tsp. olive oil

3rd Organic eggs (size M, separated)

salt

2nd Tbsp. hemp seeds (or flax seeds)

150 Milliliters (hemp drink or milk)

Pepper (freshly ground)

Nutmeg (freshly grated)

(Baking spray oil)

RAGOUT

1Onion (in cubes)

4th Tsp. olive oil

1 Tsp. marjoram (shredded)

200 Grams of mushrooms (sliced)

200 Grams of smoked tofu (cubes)

200 Grams of tomato (chopped, fresh, or canned)

sugar

3rd Tablespoons parsley (chopped, fresh or frozen)

Directions:

FLAN

Squeeze and stir up the spinach. Braise with garlic in a teaspoon of oil in a pan for about 4 minutes. Take out and let cool.

Preheat the oven to 160 degrees, convection 140 degrees, and gas level 2. Beat egg whites and a pinch of salt until stiff. Mix egg yolk, hemp seeds, hemp drink, and spinach, season with pepper, nutmeg, and salt. Carefully fold in the egg whites.

Fill the drip pan of the oven on the middle shelf approximately 2 cm high with hot water. Spray 4 cups with spray oil; distribute the spinach mixture in it. Let it set in the oven water bath for 25-30 minutes. Take out, let cool completely on a wire rack.

RAGOUT

Braise the onions in oil. Add marjoram, mushrooms, and tofu and braise. Add tomatoes, and then cook for about 8 minutes.

Season with pepper, two pinches of sugar, salt. Mix in the parsley. Arrange ragout sprinkled with two flans and hemp seeds.

Nutrition:

445 kcal,

31g fat,

11g carbohydrates,

30g protein

CHAPTER 7:

Dinner

17.   Ham Cheese And Caper Soufflé

Preparation Time: 10 minutes

Cooking Time: 30 minutes

Servings: 4

Ingredients:

Olive oil spray oil

Ham, fully cooked and diced, two cups

Garlic, minced, two tablespoons

Kale, chopped, one cup

Red onion, chopped, two tablespoons

Black pepper, one teaspoon

Greek yogurt, one half cup

Capers, two tablespoons

Cheddar cheese, low-fat, shredded, one cup

Eggs, six large

Extra virgin olive oil, two tablespoons

Directions:

Heat the oven to 400. Use the olive oil spray to grease four six-ounce ramekins or other oven-safe dishes.

 Fry the garlic, kale, and onion in the hot oil over medium heat for five minutes. Mix the diced ham, capers, cheddar cheese, onion, and garlic in a large mixing bowl.

Beat together the yogurt with the eggs and pour this over the ham mixture in the bowl. Then add the fried garlic, kale, and onion to the bowl and mix everything very well.

Divide the mixture among the oven dishes and cook them for thirty minutes.

Nutrition:

Energy (calories): 143 kcal

Protein: 4.59 g

Fat: 10.88 g

Carbohydrates: 8.03 g

18. Turmeric Chicken & Kale Salad With Honey, Lime Dressing

Preparation Time: 20 minutes

Cooking Time: 10 minutes

Servings: 2

Notes: If you are preparing before time, dress the salad 10 minutes before its serving. Also, chicken can be replaced with beef mince, chopped prawns, or fish. Vegetarians could use mushrooms or cooked quinoa.

Ingredients

Ingredients for the chicken

1teaspoon ghee or 1 tbsp. coconut oil

½ medium brown onion, diced

250-300 g / 9 oz. chicken mince or diced up chicken thighs

One large garlic clove, finely diced

One teaspoon turmeric powder

1teaspoon lime zest

juice of ½ lime

½ teaspoon salt + pepper

 For the salad

Broccolini: 6 stalks or 2 cups of broccoli florets

Pumpkin seeds (pepitas): 2 tablespoons

Three large Kale leaves stem removed, chopped

½ Avocado, slices

A handful of fresh coriander leaves, chopped

A handful of fresh parsley leaves, chopped

For the dressing

Three tablespoons lime juice

1garlic clove, finely diced or grated

small tablespoons extra-virgin olive oil (I used one tablespoon avocado oil and * 2 tablespoons EVO)

One teaspoon raw honey

½ teaspoon wholegrain or Dijon mustard

½ teaspoon sea salt and pepper

Directions:

First of all, heat the ghee or coconut oil in a small frying pan. Keep heat medium to high. Add onion and sauté on medium heat for 4-5 minutes, until they are golden. Now add chicken mince and garlic and stir for two to3 minutes over medium to high.

Now add the turmeric, lime zest, lime juice, salt, and pepper and cook them. Stir frequently, for a further 3 to 4 minutes.

Set aside the cooked mince.

While the chicken is being cooked, bring a small saucepan of water to boil. Add the broccolini to it and cook for 2 minutes. Rinse under cold water and cut into 3 to 4 pieces each.

Now add the pumpkin seeds to the frying pan from the chicken. Toast over medium heat for 2 minutes. Stir frequently to prevent burning.

Now Season with a little salt. Set it aside.

Raw pumpkin seeds are also acceptable to use.

Place the chopped kale in a salad bowl. Pour the dressing over it.

With your hands, toss and massage the kale with the sauce. It will soften the kale, like what citrus juice does to the fish or beef carpaccio as it 'cooks' it lightly.

Finally, toss it through the cooked chicken, broccolini, fresh herbs, pumpkin seeds, and avocado slices.

19. Buckwheat Noodles With Chicken, Kale & Miso Dressing

Preparation time: 15 minutes,

Cooking time: 15 minutes,

Servings: 2

Ingredients

For noodles

2-3 handfuls of kale leaves (removed from the stem and roughly cut)

150 g / 5 oz. buckwheat noodles (100% buckwheat, no wheat)

3-4 shiitake mushrooms, sliced

1teaspoon coconut oil or ghee

brown onion, finely diced

One medium free-range chicken breast, sliced or diced

One long red chili, thinly sliced (seeds in or out depending on how hot you like it)

large garlic cloves, finely diced

2-3 tablespoons Tamari sauce (gluten-free soy sauce)

For the miso dressing

1½ tablespoon fresh organic miso

One tablespoon Tamari sauce

One tablespoon extra-virgin olive oil

One tablespoon lemon or lime juice

One teaspoon sesame oil (optional)

Directions:

Bring a medium saucepan of water to boil. Add the kale and cook for 1 minute, until slightly wilted. Remove and set aside but reserve the water and bring it back to the boil. Add the soba noodles and cook according to the package instructions (usually about 5 minutes). Rinse under cold water and set aside.

Pan-fries the shiitake mushrooms in a little ghee or coconut oil (about a teaspoon) for 2-3 minutes, until lightly browned on each side. Sprinkle with sea salt and set aside.

In the same frying pan, heat more coconut oil or ghee over medium-high heat. Sauté onion and chili for 2-3 minutes, and then add the chicken pieces. Cook 5 minutes over medium heat, stirring a couple of times, then add the garlic, tamari sauce, and a little splash of water. Cook for a further 2 to 3 minutes, frequently stirring until chicken is cooked through.

Finally, add the kale and soba noodles and toss through the chicken to warm up.

Mix the miso dressing and drizzle over the noodles right at the end of cooking. This way, you will keep all those beneficial probiotics in the miso alive and active.

20. Asian King Prawns Stir-Fry With Buckwheat Noodles

Preparation Time: 10 minutes

Cooking Time: 30 minutes

Servings: 1

Ingredients

150g shelled raw king prawns, deveined

2 tsp. tamari (you can use soy sauce if you are not avoiding gluten)

2 tsp. extra virgin olive oil

75g soba (buckwheat noodles)

1garlic clove, finely chopped

One bird's eye chili, finely chopped

1 tsp. finely chopped fresh ginger

20g red onions, sliced

40g celery, trimmed and sliced

75g green beans, chopped

50g kale, roughly chopped

100ml chicken stock

5g lovage or celery leaves

Directions:

Heat frying pan over high heat. Then cook the prawns in one teaspoon of the tamari and one teaspoon of the oil for 3 minutes.

Now transfer the prawns to a plate. Wipe the pan out with kitchen paper because you're going to use it again.

Cook the noodles in boiling water for 5 to 8 minutes. Drain it. Set aside.

Now fry garlic, chili, ginger, red onion, celery, beans, and kale in the remaining oil. Cook these over medium to high heat for 2–3 minutes.

Add the stock now and bring to the boil. Simmer for a minute or two, until the vegetables are cooked but still crunchy.

Add the prawns, noodles, and lovage/celery leaves to the pan, bring back to the boil, then remove from the heat and serve.

21.   Prawn Arrabbiata

Preparation Time: 35- 40 minutes

Cooking Time: 20-30 minutes

Servings: 1

 Ingredients

125-150 g Raw or cooked prawns (Ideally king prawns)

65 g Buckwheat pasta

1tbsp Extra virgin olive oil

For arrabbiata sauce

40 g Red onion, finely chopped

1 Garlic clove, finely chopped

30 g Celery, finely chopped

1 Bird's eye chili, finely chopped

1 tsp. Dried mixed herbs

1 tsp. Extra virgin olive oil

2 tbsp. White wine (optional)

400 g Tinned chopped tomatoes

1 tbsp. Chopped parsley

Directions:

Fry the onion, garlic, celery, chili, and dried herbs in the oil over medium-low heat for 1–2 minutes. Turn the heat up to medium, add the wine, and cook for 1 minute. Add the tomatoes and leave the sauce to simmer over medium-low heat for 20–30 minutes, until it has a nice creamy consistency. If you feel the sauce is getting too thick, simply add a little water.

While the sauce is cooking, bring a pan of water to a boil, cook the pasta according to packet instructions. When cooked to your liking, drain, toss with the olive oil and keep in the pan until needed. If you are using raw prawns, add them to the sauce and cook for a further 3–4 minutes, until they have turned pink and opaque; add the parsley and serve. If you are using cooked prawns, add them with the parsley, bring the sauce to the boil, and help.

Add the cooked pasta to the sauce, mix thoroughly but gently and serve.

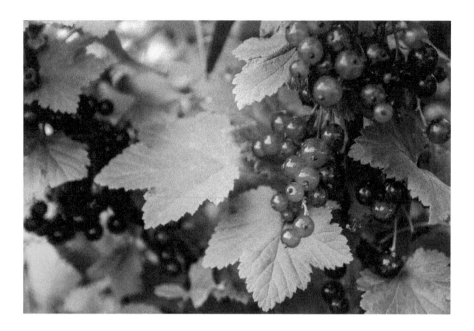

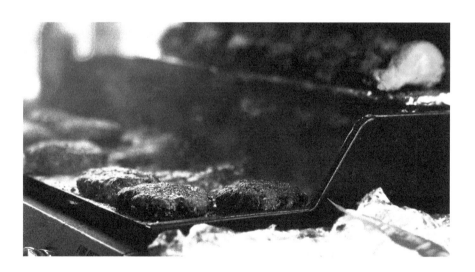

CHAPTER 8:

Mains

22.   Aromatic Chicken Breast With Tomato, Kale And Red Onions, Served With Chili Salsa

Preparation Time: 5 minutes

Cooking Time: 30 minutes

Servings: 4

Ingredients:

120g skinless, boneless chicken breast

1Tsps. ground turmeric

juice of ¼ lemon

1 tbsp. extra virgin olive oil

50g kale, chopped

20g red onion, sliced

1 tsp. chopped fresh ginger

50g buckwheat

For the salsa

130g tomato (about 1)

One bird's eye chili, finely chopped

1 tbsp. capers, finely chopped

5g parsley, finely chopped

Juice of ¼ lemon

Directions:

To prepare the salsa, cut the tomato's eye and finely slice it, make sure to retain as much liquid as possible. Pair the chili, capers, parsley, and lemon juice. You might place anything in a blender, but the end product is different.

Set the temperature of the oven up to 220°C / gas 7.

Marinate chicken breast in 1 turmeric tablespoon, lemon juice, and a little butter. Heat the frying pan until soft, then attach the marinated chicken and cook for about a minute on each side until light yellow. If your pan is not ovenproof, switch to the oven (place on the baking tray) for 8–10 minutes or until cooked through. Remove from the oven, cover with foil for 5 minutes before eating. In a steamer, cook the kale for 5 minutes. Fry the red onions and ginger in a little oil until soft but not flavored, then add the kale and fry until cooked for another minute.

Add the remaining turmeric tablespoon into the buckwheat and cook them.

Serve rice, tomatoes, and salsa.

23. Stuffed Whole-Wheat Pita

Preparation Time: 10 minutes

Cooking Time: 30 minutes

Servings: 1

Ingredients:

FOR A MEAT OPTION

cooked turkey slices, chopped 3 ounces (80g)

cheddar cheese, diced 3/4-ounce (20g)

cucumber, diced 1/4 cup (35g)

red onion, chopped 1/4 cup (35g)

arugula, chopped 1-ounce (25g)

walnuts, roughly chopped 1 1/2 to 2 tablespoons (10 to 15g)

FOR THE DRESSING

extra-virgin olive oil   1 tablespoon

balsamic vinegar 1 tablespoon

dash of lemon juice

FOR A VEGAN OPTION

hummus 2 to 3 tablespoons

cucumber, diced 1/4 cup (35g)

red onion, chopped   1/4 cup (35g)

1-ounce (25g) arugula, chopped as you like

walnuts, roughly chopped 1 1/2 to 2 tablespoons (10 to 15g)

FOR THE VEGAN DRESSING

extra-virgin olive oil 1 tablespoon

dash of lemon juice   as you like

Directions:

Entire-wheat pitas are an excellent way to pile a lot of Sirtfoods in a quick lunch or relaxing and versatile filled meal.

You can carry along and get innovative with amounts, but inevitably all you do is stack the additives in, and it's nice to go.

24. Butternut Squash And Date Tagine With Buckwheat

Preparation Time: 10 minutes

Cooking Time: 30 minutes

Servings: 4

Ingredients

extra virgin olive oil   3 teaspoons

red onion, finely sliced 1

finely sliced fresh ginger 1 tablespoon

garlic cloves, finely sliced 4

Thai chilies, finely sliced 2

ground cumin   1 tablespoon

cinnamon stick   1

ground turmeric 2 tablespoons

chopped tomatoes   2 x 14-ounce cans (400g each)

vegetable stock   1 1/4 cups (300ml)

Medjool dates, pitted and chopped 2/3 cup (100g)

of chickpeas, drained and rinsed 1 x 14-ounce can (400g)

butternut squash, peeled and cut into bite-size pieces 2 1/2 cups (500g) buckwheat 1 1/4 cups (200g)

fresh coriander, chopped 2 tablespoons (5g)

fresh parsley, chopped 1/4 cup (10g)

Directions:

Heat the oven to 400°F (200°C).

Cook the oil in 2 teaspoons with the onion, garlic, ginger, and chili for two or three minutes. Insert the cumin and cinnamon and one teaspoon of the turmeric, and then bake one to two minutes longer.

Start adding the tomatoes, stock, dates, and chickpeas, and slowly boil for 45-60 minutes. From moment to moment, you may need to insert a little more water to accomplish a thick, sticky uniformity and ensure the skillet doesn't run dry.

Put the squash in a grilling saucepan, mix with the residual oil and bake until crispy, and roast around the sides for thirty minutes.

Towards the cooking process's final moment for the tagine, fry the buckwheat with turmeric's residual spoonful as per the manufacturer guidelines.

Start adding the grilled squash and coriander, and parsley to the tagine and start serving with buckwheat.

Nutrition:Energy (calories): 2966 kcal Protein: 18.46 g Fat: 283.01 g

Carbohydrates: 126.62 g

25.   Butter Bean And Miso Dip With Celery Sticks And Oatcakes

Preparation Time: 10 minutes

Cooking Time: 0 minutes Servings: 4

Ingredients:

butter beans drained and rinsed 2 x 14-ounce cans (400g each)

extra virgin olive oil   three tablespoons

brown miso paste   two tablespoons

juice and grated zest of 1/2 unwaxed lemon   as you like

medium scallions, trimmed and finely sliced 4

garlic clove squeezed 1

Thai chili, finely sliced 1/4

celery sticks, to serve   as you like

oatcakes, to do   as you like

Directions:

Only pound the first seven components and a potato blender, and you'll have a rough combination.Start serving the celery sticks and oatcakes as a sauce.

Nutrition: Energy (calories): 213 kcal Protein: 8.17 g Fat: 8.8 g Carbohydrates: 27.79 g

26.   Yogurt With Mixed Berries, Chopped Walnuts, And Dark Chocolate

Preparation Time: 10 minutes

Cooking Time: 0 minutes

Servings: 1

Ingredients:

mixed berries   about 1 1/3 cups (125g)

plain Greek yogurt (or vegan alternative, such as soy or coconut yogurt) 2/3 cup (150g)

walnuts, chopped 1/4 cup (25g)

dark chocolate (85 percent cocoa solids), grated   1   1/2 tablespoons (10g)

Directions:

Just add your favorite berries to a pot and upper surface with the yogurt.

Spray with the dark chocolates and the walnuts.

27. Chicken And Kale Curry With Bombay Potatoes

Preparation Time: 10 minutes

Cooking Time: 90 minutes

Servings: 4

Ingredients:

skinless, boneless chicken breasts, cut into bite-size pieces 4 x 4 ½ - to 5 ½ -ounce (120 to 150g)

extra virgin olive oil   4 tablespoons

ground turmeric 3 tablespoons

red onions, sliced 2

Thai chilies, finely sliced 2

garlic cloves, finely sliced 3

finely sliced fresh ginger 1 tablespoon

mild curry powder 1 tablespoon

can chopped tomatoes 1 x 14-ounce (400g)

chicken stock 2 1/8 cups (500ml)

coconut milk 7/8 cup (200ml)

cardamom pods 2

cinnamon stick   1

russet potatoes   1 1/3 pounds (600g)

parsley, chopped 1/4 cup (10g)

kale, chopped   2 2/3 cups (175g)

coriander, chopped   2 tablespoons (5g)

Directions:

Massage the chicken breast in one teaspoon of oil and one tablespoon of turmeric. Mean leaving on for thirty min to marinate.

Roast the meat over high temperature (the meat should be fried with adequate oil in the marinade) for four to five minutes just until golden brown all over it and fried completely, then remove from heat and cast aside.

Start heating one spoonful of the oil over the moderate flame in the roasting pan and insert the onion, chili, garlic, and ginger. Roast for about ten minutes till soft, then introduce the curry powder and then another turmeric spoonful and prepare food for more than one to two minutes. Append the tomatoes to the pan and allow roasting for another two min. Include the stock, coconut milk, cardamom, and cinnamon stick and left for forty-five to sixty minutes to boil. Inspect the pan frequently to make sure it doesn't dry up — you may need to insert more storage.

Heat the oven to 425 ° F (220 ° C). Scrape the potatoes as your gravy is cooking, then slice them into smaller pieces. Put the residual teaspoon of turmeric in boiling water, and simmer for five minutes. Flush well and permit for ten minutes of dry steam. Round every edge, they must be white and waxy.

Move to a baking dish, mix in the residual oil, and grill till nicely browned and crunchy after 30 minutes. When the recipe is fully prepared, throw the parsley across. nsert the kale, roasted chicken, and coriander when the sauce has your optimum requirements, roast for another five minutes to make sure the meat is cooked across, and then start serving with the potatoes.

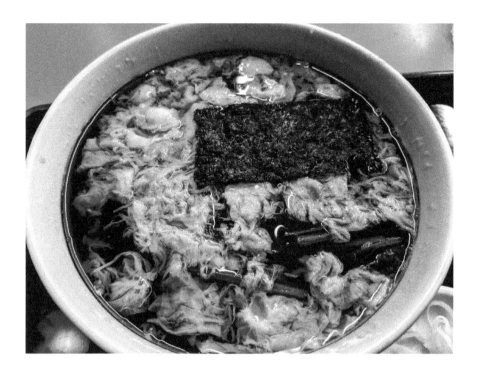

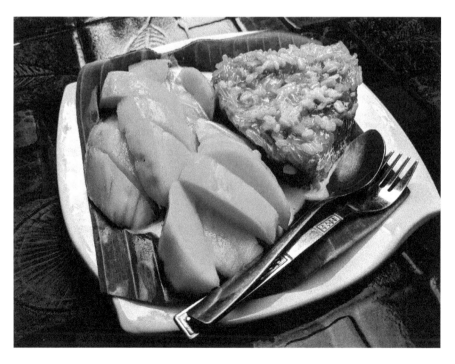

CHAPTER 9:

Meat

28.   Sirtfood Lamb

Ingredients:

2 tbsp. Extra virgin olive oil

Grated ginger, one inch

One sliced red onion.

1 tsp. of bird's eye

Cumin seeds 2 tsp.

One cinnamon stick

Lamb, 800 g

Garlic cloves, crushed, three pieces

A pinch of salt

Chopped Medjool dates, 1 cup

Chickpeas, 400 g

Coriander, 2 tbsp.

Buckwheat

Directions:

Start by preheating your oven to 140 °C. Sauté sliced onion with 2 tbsp. Of extra virgin olive oil for five minutes while keeping the lid on. The onions should turn soft but not brown.

Add turmeric, cumin, ginger, garlic, and chili and stir fry for another minute.

Add the chunks of lamb, season with salt and let, and let boil. Add a glass of water.

After the mixture has boiled, roast in the oven for one hour and 15 minutes. Add the chickpeas half an hour before the dish are finished.

Add chopped coriander and serve with buckwheat after the meal is done.

Nutrition:

Energy (calories): 199 kcal

Protein: 1.6 g

Fat: 13g

Carbohydrates: 21.72 g

CHAPTER 10:

Sides

29. Broccoli Stew

Preparation Time: 10 minutes.

Cooking Time: 40 minutes

Servings: 4

Ingredients:

One broccoli head, separated into florets

2 tsp. coriander seeds

The drizzle of olive oil

One onion, peeled and chopped

Salt and ground black pepper to taste

A pinch of red pepper, crushed

One small ginger piece, peeled and chopped

One garlic clove, peeled and minced

28-oz. can have pureed tomatoes

Directions:

Put water in a pot, add the salt, bring to a boil over medium-high heat, add the broccoli florets, steam them for 2 minutes, transfer them to a bowl filled with ice water, drain them, and set aside.

Heat a pan over medium-high heat, add the coriander seeds, toast them for 4 minutes, transfer to a grinder, grind them, and set aside as well. Heat a pot with the oil over medium heat, add the onions, salt, pepper, and red pepper, stir, and cook for 7 minutes.

Add the ginger, garlic, and coriander seeds, stir and cook for 3 minutes. Add the tomatoes, bring to a boil, and simmer for 10 minutes. Add the broccoli, stir, and cook the stew for 12 minutes.

Divide into bowls and serve.

Nutrition: Calories 150 Fat 4 g Carbs 5 g Protein 12 g

30.   Collard Greens And Tomatoes

Preparation Time: 10 minutes.

Cooking Time: 12 minutes

Servings: 5

Ingredients:

1-pound collard greens

Three bacon strips, chopped

¼ cup cherry tomatoes, halved

1 tbsp. apple cider vinegar

2 tbsp. chicken stock

Salt and ground black pepper to taste

Directions:

Heat a pan over medium heat, add the bacon, stir, and cook until it browns. Add the tomatoes, collard greens, vinegar, stock, salt, and pepper, stir and cook for 8 minutes.

Add more salt and pepper, stir again gently, divide onto plates, and serve.

Nutrition: Calories 120 Fat 8 g Carbs 3 g Protein 7 g

31.   Roasted Radishes

Preparation Time: 10 minutes.

Cooking Time: 35 minutes

Servings: 2

Ingredients:

2 cups radishes cut in quarters

Salt and ground black pepper to taste

2 tbsp. butter, melted

1 tbsp. fresh chives, chopped

1 tbsp. lemon zest

Directions:

Spread the radishes on a lined baking sheet. Add the salt, pepper, chives, lemon zest, and butter, toss to coat, and bake in the oven at 375°F for 35 minutes.

Divide onto plates and serve.

Nutrition:

 Calories 122 Fat 12 g Carbs 3 g Protein 14 g

CHAPTER 11:

Seafood

32.   Salmon Super Sirt Salad

Preparation time: 25 minutes

Cooking time: 0 minutes

Servings: 4

Ingredients:

50g chicory leaves

100g smoked salmon slices (you can also use lentils, cooked chicken breast, or tinned tuna)

80g avocado, peeled, stoned, and sliced

40g celery, sliced

20g red onion, sliced

15g walnuts, chopped

One tbs. capers

One large Medjool date, pitted and chopped

One tbs. extra-virgin olive oil

Juice ¼ lemon

10g parsley, chopped

10g lovage or celery leaves, chopped

Directions:

Arrange the salad leaves beautifully on a large plate or bowl.

Mix all the remaining ingredients and serve on top of the leaves

CHAPTER 12:

Poultry

33.   Chicken Radicchio And Turmeric

Preparation time: 10 minutes

Cooking time: 25 minutes

Servings: 4

Ingredients

350 g basmati rice

200 g chicken meat

One small onion

One red pepper

1 liter of vegetable stock

Four cardamom seeds

1/2 teaspoon of turmeric

chili pepper

Evo oil

halls

chives

Directions:

Pour the turmeric into half a glass of boiling water.

Fry the onion cut into three tablespoons of oil, add the cardamom seeds, the pepper cut into small pieces, and the turmeric water. Let it cook for five minutes. Cut the chicken into pieces and add it to the pan with the peppers. After a few regular minutes of salt, add the chili pepper and stir.

Boil the basmati rice in vegetable stock for about 9 minutes. Drain the excess water, arrange the rice on plates and place the chicken and pepper seasoning in the center. Decorate with chives, finish with a drizzle of oil

CHAPTER 13:

Vegetable

34.   Artichoke Petals Bites

Preparation Time: 10 minutes

Cooking time: 10 minutes

Servings:8

Ingredients:

8 oz artichoke petals, boiled, drained, without salt

½ cup almond flour

4 oz Parmesan, grated

2 tablespoons almond butter, melted

Directions: In the mixing bowl, mix up together almond flour and grated Parmesan. Preheat the oven to 355F. Dip the artichoke petals in the almond butter and then coat in the almond flour mixture. Place them in the tray. Transfer the tray in the preheated oven and cook the petals for 10 minutes. Chill the cooked petal bites little before serving.

Nutrition: calories 140, fat 6.4, fiber 7.6, carbs 14.6, protein 10

35.   Rutabaga Latkes

Preparation Time: 15 minutes

Cooking time: 7 minutes

Servings:4

Ingredients:

1 teaspoon hemp seeds

1 teaspoon ground black pepper

7 oz rutabaga, grated

½ teaspoon ground paprika

2 tablespoons coconut flour

1 egg, beaten

1 teaspoon olive oil

Directions:

Mix up together hemp seeds, ground black pepper, ground paprika, and coconut flour.

Then add grated rutabaga and beaten egg.

With the help of the fork combine together all the ingredients into the smooth mixture.

Preheat the skillet for 2-3 minutes over the high heat.

Then reduce the heat till medium and add olive oil.

With the help of the fork, place the small amount of rutabaga mixture in the skillet. Flatten it gently in the shape of latkes.

Cook the latkes for 3 minutes from each side.

After this, transfer them in the plate and repeat the same steps with remaining rutabaga mixture.

Nutrition: calories 64, fat 3.1, fiber 3, carbs 7.1, protein 2.8

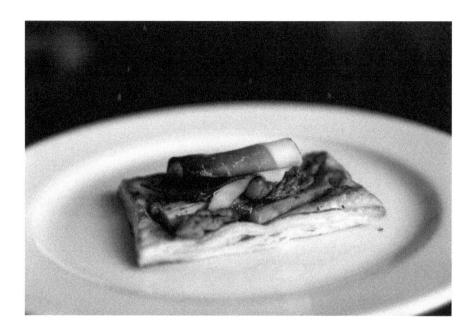

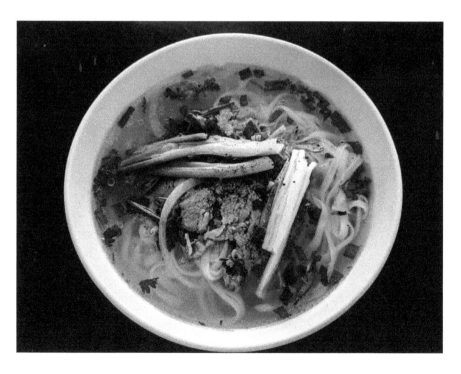

CHAPTER 14:

Soup, Curries and Stews

36.   Palak Daal - Kale Lentil Stew

Preparation Time: 10 minutes Cooking Time: 7-9 hours

Servings:8

Ingredients:

3 cups kale, chopped

1 cup curry paste

3 Tbsp. olive oil

2 cups chopped onions & 2 cloves minced garlic

3 cups dried lentils

Salt & 1 Tsp. ground pepper to taste

4 cups water

1 Tsp. red pepper flakes 2 Tbsp. lemon juice

Directions:

Put ingredients in the slow cooker.Cover, and cook on low for 7 to 9 hours.

37.   Ewedu – Modified Nigerian Kale Stew

Preparation Time: 10 minutes

Cooking Time: 7-9 hours

Servings:8

Ingredients:

4 cups mallow leaves – optionally 4 cups kale – blended if you want

2 cups chopped red onions & 2 cloves minced garlic

2 cups sliced mushrooms

3 Tbsp. olive oil

Salt & 1 Tsp. ground pepper to taste

1 Tsp. red pepper flakes

2 cups fish broth

3 pounds shrimp

Direction:

 Put ingredients in the slow cooker. Cover, and cook on low for 7 to 9 hours.

38.   Lentil Kale Stew

Preparation Time: 10 minutes

Cooking Time: 7-9 hours

Servings: 8

Ingredients:

2 cups chopped onions

2 tbsp. olive oil

3 cups chopped Kale

3 tomatoes

Salt, ground black pepper, and ground cumin to taste

3 cups beef stock

4 cups dry lentils

Direction:

Put ingredients in the slow cooker. Cover, and cook on low for 7 to 9 hours

39.   Roast Chicken With Arugula

Preparation Time: 10 minutes

Cooking Time: 30 minutes

Servings: 6-8

Ingredients:

1 (3 pounds) whole chicken, rinsed, skinned

Salt and pepper to taste

1 red onion, quartered

1/4 cup chopped rosemary

2 cups arugula

Directions

Heat the oven to 350F. Sprinkle salt and pepper on the meat—stuff with the onion and rosemary.

Place in a baking dish and bake in the preheated oven until chicken is cooked through. Depending on the size of the bird, cooking time will vary. Serve on a bed of arugula.

Nutrition:

Energy (calories): 81 kcal

Protein: 3.37 g Fat: 0.86g

Carbohydrates: 17.4 g

CHAPTER 15:

Snacks & Desserts

40. Greek Salad Skewers-Sirt Food Recipes

Preparation Time: 5 minutes

Cooking Time: 25 minutes

Servings: 4

Ingredients:

306 Energy • 3.5 of One's SIRT 5 per day

Serves 2 • All Set at ten moments

Two wooden skewers, soaked in plain water for 30 minutes earlier. Utilize

Eight big black olives

Eight cherry tomatoes

One yellow pepper, cut into eight squares

1/2 reddish onion, then cut and separated into 8 bits

100g (roughly 10cm) cucumber, cut into four pieces, and simmer

100g feta, cut into eight cubes

For Your dressing:

One tablespoon extra-virgin olive oil

Taste of 1/2 lemon

One teaspoon balsamic vinegar

1/2 teaspoons garlic, crushed and peeled

A handful of leaves basil, finely chopped (or even 1/2 teaspoon dried blended Herbaceous plants to displace peppermint and eucalyptus)

A handful of leaves eucalyptus, thinly sliced

The generous flavor of salt and freshly ground black pepper

Directions:

Inch tsp. Each skewer using all the salad components at the Order: tomato, olive, yellow pepper, red onion, cucumber, feta, olive, tomato oil, yellow pepper, red onion, cucumber, feta.

2 Put all of the dressing ingredients in a little bowl and then blend thoroughly. Pour the skewers.

41. Fruity Granola Bars

Preparation time: 25 minutes

Cooking Time: 15 Minutes

Servings: 24 Bars

Ingredients

¾ cup packed brown sugar

½ cup honey

¼ cup of water

1teaspoon salt

½ cup of cocoa butter

3cups rolled oats

1cup walnuts, chopped

1cup ground buckwheat

¼ cup sesame seeds

½ cup dried strawberries or mixed fruits

½ cup raisins

½ cup Medjool dates, chopped

Directions

In a large pan, combine sugar, cocoa butter, honey, water, and salt. Bring to a simmer and cook for 5 minutes. Stir in oats, walnuts, ground buckwheat, and sesame seeds. Cook, frequently stirring, for 15 minutes. Remove from heat and add dried fruits. Pour into a large baking sheet lined with wax or parchment paper. ress firmly to create an even layer. Score deeply into bars roughly 2" wide by 4" tall. Allow cooling for 30 minutes before breaking or cutting along score lines. Store in an airtight container.

Nutrition:

Calorie: 441

Fat: 17.5

Carbs: 59.1

Sodium: 257

Protein: 8.7

42.   Tortilla Chips And Fresh Salsa

Preparation time: 10 minutes

Cooking Time: 10 Minutes

Servings: 4

Ingredients

Four whole wheat flour tortillas

Two tablespoons extra virgin olive oil

4 Roma tomatoes, diced

1small red onion, finely diced

1 Bird's Eye chili pepper, finely diced

Two teaspoons parsley, finely chopped

Two teaspoons cilantro, finely chopped

1lime, juiced

Salt and pepper to taste

Directions

Preheat oven to 350 degrees F. using a pastry brush, coat one side of each tortilla in olive oil. A sharp knife or pizza cutter divides each tortilla into eight wedges—spread tortillas over a large baking sheet in a single layer. Use more than one baking sheet if necessary. Bake for 8 – 10 minutes, flipping halfway through until both sides are golden brown and your chips are crispy. While the chips are baking, combine tomatoes, red onion, chili pepper, parsley, cilantro, and lime juice and mix well. Serve salsa with the chips.

Nutrition:

Calorie: 375 Fat: 19 g

Carbs: 47 g Sodium: 215 mg

Protein: 5g

43. Garlic Baked Kale Chips

Preparation time: 30 minutes

Cooking Time: 25 Minutes

Servings: 4

Ingredients

1bunch kale leaves

½ tablespoon extra-virgin olive oil

1teaspoon garlic powder

1/8 teaspoon cayenne powder

¼ teaspoon fine salt

Directions

Preheat oven to 300 degrees F and cover a large baking sheet with parchment paper. Remove the stems from your kale and tear up into large pieces.

Wash and spin the leaves until thoroughly dry, using a paper towel to pat dry if necessary.

Place kale leaves in a large bowl and massage the olive oil thoroughly into each plate.

Combine garlic, cayenne, and salt in a small bowl and mix well. Sprinkle seasoning over kale and toss to distribute.

Spread the kale in a single layer over the baking sheet.

Bake for 10 minutes, rotate the pan, and bake for another 12-15 minutes more until the kale just begins to get crispy. The leaves will shrink and need to cool at least 5 minutes after being taken out of the oven to crisp properly.

Nutrition:

Calorie: 108 kcal

Fat: 9

Carbs: 4

Sodium: 49

Protein: 2

CHAPTER 16:

Desserts

44.   Chocolate Cake Without Flour

Preparation Time: 10 minutes

Cooking Time: 40 minutes

Servings: 4

Ingredients

125 g dark chocolate (70% cocoa content)

100 g butter

150 g cane sugar

3 eggs (l)

40 g cocoa powder

cocoa powder for dusting

Directions:

Roughly chop the chocolate and melt it with the butter in a bowl over a hot but not boiling water bath, stirring occasionally.

Remove from the heat and stir the sugar into the chocolate.

Whisk the eggs lightly and stir into the chocolate.

Mix in the cocoa powder.

Put everything in a springform pan covered with baking paper (20 cm Ø) and knock it flat.

Bake the cake in the preheated oven at 180 ° C (forced air 160 ° C, gas: level 2–3) for 25–30 minutes.

 Remove from the oven and let cool in the tin for 5 minutes.

Open the springform pan; remove the cake from the edge of the mold with a knife. Carefully put the cake on a plate.

Mix the icing sugar and cocoa powder and sprinkle with the cake.

Nutrition:

Energy (calories): 2115 kcal

Protein: 43.68 g

Fat: 164.51 g

Carbohydrates: 119.51 g

45. Chicory And Orange Salad

Preparation Time: 10 minutes

Cooking Time: 50 minutes

Servings: 4

Ingredients

Two chicory

Two oranges

1 tsp. honey

1 tbsp. light vinegar, e.g., B. white balsamic vinegar

Two tablespoons of walnut oil

Salt and pepper

at will walnut kernels

Directions:

Wash the chicory and cut into rough strips.Fillets of 1.5 oranges squeeze out the remaining half of the orange.Mix the orange juice, honey, vinegar, oil, salt, and pepper generously.Add chicory and orange fillets and let steep for half an hour. Sprinkle with chopped walnut kernels as desired.

Nutrition:Energy (calories): 161 kcal Protein: 0.69 g Fat: 13.75 g Carbohydrates: 10.32 g

46.   Mango And Avocado Salad With Watercress

Preparation Time: 10 minutes

Cooking Time: 20 minutes

Servings: 4

Ingredients

Salad:

Three handfuls of watercress (approx. 150 g)

One mango

One avocado

One spring onion

2 tbsp. coriander leaves

A little lime juice (lemon juice is, of course, also possible)

Dressing:

Two cloves of garlic, finely diced

2/3 tsp. ginger, finely diced

3 tbsp. light sesame oil

One tablespoon of rice vinegar

Salt and pepper

Some brown sugar

One chili pepper without seeds, amount depending on the spiciness and taste, very finely diced

a little dark sesame oil

Directions:

Salad:

Clean, wash, spin dry watercress, and cut it into bite-size pieces.

Peel the mango and avocado, remove the stones, and cut the pulp into wedges. Immediately drizzle the avocado with a little lime juice so that it doesn't turn brown.

Clean, wash, and cut the spring onions into thin rings.

Pluck coriander leaves a little smaller depending on the size.

Dressing:

Sweat the garlic and ginger in half a tablespoon of heated light sesame oil, place in a bowl and let cool.

Mix in the vinegar, salt, pepper, and sugar.

Fold in the remaining light oil.

Add the chili to taste.

Season with the dark sesame oil.

47. White Chocolate And Pistachio Cookies

Preparation Time: 10 minutes

Cooking Time: 30 minutes

Servings: 4

Ingredients:

100 g butter at room temperature

200 g of sugar

1medium egg

5 g of baking powder

200 g of flour

125 g of white chocolate

30 g pistachios

Directions:

Put the butter at room temperature, sugar, flour, and yeast in a bowl. Work the mixture well with your hands until you get the consistency of some crumbs. Next, the egg is added and integrated without kneading. Let the dough rest a little.

Meanwhile, chocolate and peeled pistachios are chopped and added to the mixture by gently kneading. When everything is already bound, let the dough rest in the fridge for at least an hour.

Preheat the oven to 190° C. Take small portions of dough and give the cookies' desired shape. Bake on a tray with baking paper for 9 minutes and let them cool on a rack.

Nutrition

130 kcal

9.2 g of fat

3.2 g of carbohydrates

9.2 g of protein

48.   Chocolate Biscuits With Vanilla Cream Recipe

Preparation Time: 10 minutes

Cooking Time: 30 minutes

Servings: 4

Ingredients:

50 g of cover chocolate

50 g of nuts (nuts, almonds, hazelnuts)

1egg

50 g butter - 85 g flour

50 g brown sugar

For the vanilla cream:

1egg yolk

30 g of sugar

100 ml whole milk

One vanilla pod

Directions:

Shell the egg and incorporate it in a bowl with the whole sugar. Beat with the rod blender and add the butter. Mix well and add the flour and chocolate topping. Stir, chop the nuts very fine with a knife (nuts, almonds, and hazelnuts), incorporate them, and mix everything with a spatula until you make a compact chocolate dough.

Make balls with the chocolate dough (16) and place them on a baking sheet covered with baking paper. The balls are shaped like a cookie; place another baking paper on them, and crush them by hand. Bake at 180 ° C for 15 minutes and remove.

To make the vanilla cream, heat the milk in a saucepan (reserve a little in a bowl) with the sugar. Open the vanilla bean, remove the seeds and add them to the saucepan along with the two halves of the vanilla bean. Add the egg yolk to the milk reserved in the bowl. Pour the vanilla-scented milk into this bowl, mix and put the cream back into the saucepan. Stir with a rod, simmer, and reserve.

Serve the cookies on the plate and accompany with the vanilla cream incorporated in two glasses. Decorate the cream with the vanilla bean split in two.

Nutrition

4%Total Carbohydrates 11ggrams

8%Dietary Fiber 2ggrams

Sugars 7ggrams

Protein 7g

49.   Chocolate And Blueberry Cookie Recipe

Preparation Time: 10 minutes

Cooking Time: 35 minutes

Servings: 4

Ingredients:

75 gr of butter

100 gr of sugar

1egg

140 gr of milk chocolate

170 gr of flour

5 gr of chemical yeast (baking powders)

60 gr of dried cranberries

mint leaves

Directions:

Place the sugar and butter (at room temperature) in a bowl and beat with the electric rod. When it begins to bleach, add the egg and continue beating until it is integrated. Add the blueberries and mix well.

Melt the chocolate (in the microwave or the water bath) and add it to the previous mixture. Sift the flour and yeast and incorporate them. Mix with smooth and enveloping movements.

Line 2 baking sheets with baking paper. Take small portions of dough and spread them on the baking sheets—Bake at 180 ° C for 20 minutes.

Take them out of the oven, let them cool, and place them in a bowl. Garnish with mint leaves. Serve the chocolate and blueberry cookies.

Nutrition:

This dessert gives us the total sugar recommended for one day. They are energy cookies recommended for people with excellent physical wear, such as athletes. However, they are not recommended for people with cholesterol and overweight, although it all depends on the number of cookies consumed.

We will accompany them with a glass of milk to avoid excessive consumption of cookies, complete the nutritional value of dessert, and reduce cookies' glycemic index.

50. Recipe For Cereal And Pine Nuts Cookies

Preparation Time: 10 minutes

Cooking Time: 40 minutes

Servings: 12 cookies

Ingredients:

200 g of mixed cereal flakes (oatmeal, spelled, barley)

125 g butter

120 g brown sugar

11 g yeast

50 g of pine nuts

1egg

1lemon

Mint

Directions:

Beat the egg inside a bowl; add sugar, yeast, cereal flakes. Grate the lemon peel and add it. Mix well.

Put the butter in a bowl, FUNDELA in the microwave, and incorporate it into the mixture above. Add the pine nuts and stir gently.

Take small portions of dough and distribute them in the molds.

Preheat the oven and introduce the cookies. Bake it at 180 ° C for roughly 20-25 minutes. Garnish with mint and serve the cereal and pine nut cookies.

Advice:

It is advisable to keep them in a tightly sealed jar or box to protect cookies from moisture.

Nutrition:

They are healthy cookies that can be nutritious breakfasts or snacks, especially for people who make significant physical efforts, athletes, children, and low-weight people.

51.   Chocolate Butter Cookies Recipe

Preparation Time: 10 minutes

Cooking Time: 30 minutes

Servings: 12

Ingredients:

150 grams of butter

100 grams of sugar (½ cup)

1egg

250 grams of flour

One teaspoon vanilla essence

One handful of chocolate chips

Directions:

Soften butter for a few seconds in the microwave to be easily mixed (EYE: it does not have to be liquid, only soft, if it is at room temperature, it does not need to be heated). Place it in a bowl and beat it with the sugar. Then, add the egg and vanilla essence.

Trick: If you don't have vanilla essence to add to the chocolate butter cookie mix, you can also grate a little vanilla on the branch.

Then continue mixing and, little by little, add the flour. Take the dough and make a ball. Once the shape is done, wrap it with plastic wrap and leave it for about an hour in the refrigerator.

Trick: If you see the flour sticks, the right solution is to wet your hands with water and sprinkle some flour.

When ready, go kneading until left with a thickness of about half a centimeter. Here you can put the chocolate chips or sprinkles, crushing them with the roller to integrate well into the dough. As we said at the beginning, you can make the seeds yourself. Instead, you want to try to make them with white chocolate and do not miss our "White Chocolate Cookie Recipe."

Then, cut the cookies any way you want; if you have molds to make the butter and chocolate cookies easily, better.

If not, you can improvise figures with a knife, or you can simply use the round mouth of a glass.

Trick: If you do not have a mold for the shape of cookies, you can also place them with the help of a spoon or form them with the palm of your hands.

Finally, preheat the oven to 180 ° C and carefully put the cookies on a nonstick baking sheet (or simply put flour sprinkled on the baking sheet). Bake the homemade cookies for 10 to 15 minutes, or until you see that they are golden brown.

Let cool and enjoy these chocolate butter cookies!

Homemade Chocolate Butter Cookies - Tricks

Baking some homemade cookies of envy is sometimes not as easy as it seems in recipes. The dough can stick, or cookies lose shape. They may be too crunchy or too soft. The balance between the ingredients may not be to the point. Do not be discouraged! With practice and some tricks, indeed, your butter cookies with chocolate will be perfect.

First of all, it is essential to follow a good recipe that helps you find the ideal flavor.

You can stroll through some of our recipes, such as chocolate-filled butter cookies or cream-and-butter cookies, so that you can try the best options.

On the other hand, you must wait for the cookie dough to cool to stretch and knead it.

The roller can stick if you do it at room temperature, and it will be harder for you to reach the dough's ideal thickness.

Finally, do not forget to preheat the oven to cook your butter and chocolate cookies evenly.

However, before preheating it, remove the plate from the oven so that once you insert the cookies, the tray is at room temperature and helps the cookies maintain their shape.

With these tips, you will indeed become an expert on homemade cookies. You'll see how easy it is!And if you feel like trying some cookies with more chocolate flavor, check out this other recipe: "Homemade chocolate cookies."

NutritionCarbs 83 g Dietary Fiber 4 g Sugar 66 g Protein 4 g

Conclusions

Most diets have been proven to be just a temporary fix. If you want to keep weight off for a good while maintaining muscle mass and ensuring that your body stays healthy, then you need to be following a diet that activates your sirtuin genes: in other words, the Sirtfood Diet.

Sirtuins play an essential role in burning body fat and also help to increase the metabolic rate. But sirtuin genes aren't just responsible for weight loss and muscle gain—they also help prevent illnesses such as heart disease, diabetes, bone problems, Alzheimer's, and even cancer. To activate these genes, you must eat foods that are high in the plant-based proteins polyphenols. These are known as sirtfoods and include kale and walnuts and drinks such as green tea and red wine.